I'M A NURSE WHO HELPED CURE CANCER

Cover Designer: Angela Milam

Editor: Angela Milam

Typesetter: Angela Milam

Angel Publishing Company, LLC

111 Princess Ann Drive

Macon, Georgia 31211

(478) 952-3520

www.angelpublingcompany.com

Publisher's Cataloging-in-Publication Data

I'M A NURSE WHO HELPED CURE MY METASTIC CANCER

Names: Milam, Angela, 1968, Author

Title: I'm A Nurse Who Helped Cure My Metastatic Cancer, Angela Milam, RN

Description: A short descriptive narrative of the alternative treatment used to help cure my cancer

Macon, GA: Angel Publishing Company

ISBN 979-8-9883560-3-5

Subject: An Alternative Cure for My Metastatic Cancer

Copyright © 2025 by Angela Milam

I'M A NURSE WHO HELPED CURE MY METASTIC CANCER

All rights reserved. No part of this publication may be reproduced, scanned, uploaded, stored in a retrieval system, or transmitted, in any form or by any means, electronic, mechanical, photocopying, recording, or otherwise, without the prior written permission of the publisher.

Printed in the United States of America

I'M A NURSE WHO HELPED CURE MY METASTIC CANCER

Hello, thank you for purchasing my book. I made this book short and to the point on purpose because simply people who are sick are busy trying to get cured and doesn't feel like reading dozens of pages to figure out how. I am not a doctor; I am a Registered Nurse in Georgia. I was diagnosed with breast cancer (triple negative Stage 3 Grade 3) with metastasis in three areas in August of 2020. I done extensive research and reading after receiving my

I'M A NURSE WHO HELPED CURE MY METASTIC CANCER

diagnosis. I did do traditional treatment (chemotherapy and radiation) even though I did not finish either one of them simply because they were just too harsh on me. If I had it do over again, I would have skipped the radiation. It's been four years since I've had the radiation and I'm still burning and hurting from it. I've also developed neuropathy in my hands and feet from the chemotherapy. I was diagnosed with

I'M A NURSE WHO HELPED CURE MY METASTIC CANCER

fibromyalgia after treatments as well.

I am going to go ahead and get to the good part.

The first thing I took was vitamin B17 with Amygdalin- 600mg daily. The only place I could find it was a distributor on eBay. It costs about $60 a bottle. I found out about B17 from Oasis of Hope Hospital in Tijuana, Mexico. This is a world renown cancer hospital that people with stage 3 and stage 4 cancer go to for treatment.

I'M A NURSE WHO HELPED CURE MY METASTIC CANCER

People from all over the world go there for treatment. If you read their reviews on Google you will see mostly 5-star reviews but there are some bad reviews as well like any other place. This book is only to inform you of what helped cure me. I have seen some posts on Google about B17 not being legit and being a poison. Chemotherapy is poison. It kills good cells and sometimes kills the patient and if you have an honest oncologist like I did, they will

I'M A NURSE WHO HELPED CURE MY METASTIC CANCER

tell you that. Yes, B17 with Amygdalin has apricot seeds in it which is what helps kill your cancer. I took it for over a year. I will not hide it; it converts to cyanide but that is why you only take the amount of 600mg a day. This is a controlled therapeutic dose. The cancer hospital in Tijuana, Mexico uses this vitamin in treating patients with many types of Stage 4 cancers. Jason Winters also took the B17 as well as his herbal tea. I read his book, "The Jason Winters Story".

I'M A NURSE WHO HELPED CURE MY METASTIC CANCER

The next thing I did was drank Jason Winters Tea with Chaparral. You can buy this online at www.sirjasonwinterstea.com. It's about $12.99 a box and they run specials often. Sometimes you can buy one box and get one free or buy two boxes and get 1 free. You need to drink one cup before each meal and one at bedtime. If you don't eat three meals a day, then drink the tea before you do eat and then at bedtime, but at least get in two cups a day. If

> I'M A NURSE WHO HELPED CURE MY METASTIC CANCER

you get the teabags, boil one cup of water and then pour the boiled water in a coffee cup, put the teabag in it and let it steep for 15-20 minutes. Take a spoon and gently press the teabag against the cup to get more of the herbs out. You can add a little honey if you want to sweeten it. Drink up. ☺

Ok, we can't talk about cancer cures without talking about your diet. First and foremost, the number one superfood is **broccoli**. Eat

> I'M A NURSE WHO HELPED CURE MY METASTIC CANCER

some raw broccoli daily. How much broccoli? At least two cups. Do NOT boil it. If you absolutely cannot eat it raw then you can steam it lightly. If you want to season it that's ok or add some dressing. Eat at least one clove of **garlic daily**. I ate two. I sauteed mine in a little bit of real butter.

Juice enough of organic carrots to drink **one cup of carrot juice daily**. If you absolutely cannot find organic carrots then at least

I'M A NURSE WHO HELPED CURE MY METASTIC CANCER

get the carrots you can find. There are other cancer fighting foods you should be incorporating in your diet.

HERE'S A LIST:

Brussels Sprouts

(Not boiled-preferably steamed or baked, great cut in half with a few bacon bits)

Cherries (not the kind in the jar)

Coffee

Cauliflower

(Preferably steamed)

I'M A NURSE WHO HELPED CURE MY METASTIC CANCER

Cranberries

Apples

Asparagus

(sauteed in real butter or olive oil is very good)

Blueberries

Flaxseed

Grapefruit

Grapes-red

Kale

(raw with a little dressing is best)

Oranges

I'M A NURSE WHO HELPED CURE MY METASTIC CANCER

Dry beans and peas

(boiled until done with seasoning of your choice)

Lentils

Raspberries

Soy

Spinach

(raw is best or sauteed in real butter or olive oil)

Any type of Winter Squash

Strawberries

Tomatoes

Walnuts

I'M A NURSE WHO HELPED CURE MY METASTIC CANCER

Sweet Potatoes

Whole wheat flour

Bulgur

Oatmeal

(may add a hint of brown sugar, cinnamon and real butter)

Brown rice

Quinoa

Buckwheat

Barley

Popcorn (one of my favorites)

Whole-wheat pasta

I'M A NURSE WHO HELPED CURE MY METASTIC CANCER

Turmeric

Reduce red and processed meats, alcohol, smoking and sugar

I told you this was going to be short and to the point. Use your food list to shop with. Order your B17 and tea as soon as possible.

> I'M A NURSE WHO HELPED CURE MY METASTIC CANCER

DISCLAIMER: No information in this book is **promised** to cure cancer or prolong life. It is for informational purposes only. Any products suggested or bought will be taken at your own risk.

SOME CANCER RECIPES FOR YOU

I'M A NURSE WHO HELPED CURE MY METASTIC CANCER

Kale salad with quinoa and roasted sweet potatoes

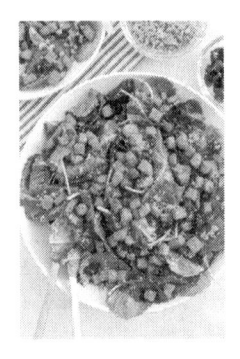

4 cups kale chopped; stems removed

1 cup cooked quinoa

1 large sweet potato peeled & cubed

3 tablespoons olive oil

I'M A NURSE WHO HELPED CURE MY METASTIC CANCER

1/2 teaspoon paprika

Salt and Pepper to taste

1 clove garlic minced

2 tablespoons lemon juice

1 teaspoon Dijon mustard

Preheat oven to 400 F (200C) Mix sweet potatoes in olive oil salt and pepper and cook on a pan for 20-25 minutes or until tender.

Add Kale and Quinoa and remaining ingredients together and stir several times. When potatoes are done add to mixture and stir.

I'M A NURSE WHO HELPED CURE MY METASTIC CANCER

Pasta Primavera

A great way to incorporate a variety of different vegetables into the dish.

Sauté a colorful mix of vegetables like zucchini, bell peppers, broccoli, spinach, and asparagus in olive oil, and toss them with the cooked whole wheat pasta.

You can add some grilled chicken or shrimp for extra

> I'M A NURSE WHO HELPED CURE MY METASTIC CANCER

protein (I grab a pack of boneless skinless chicken and chop it into chunks, then add your favorite seasoning for some seriously amazing chicken). Need a quicker version? Grab a rotisserie chicken and chop it up.

Finish with a sprinkle of Parmesan cheese, lemon and fresh basil for a bursting with flavor.

Chicken Fajitas

> I'M A NURSE WHO HELPED CURE MY METASTIC CANCER

Chicken fajitas are a quick and easy dinner option that's packed with flavor. Sauté strips of chicken breast with bell peppers and onions in a mix of chili powder, cumin, and paprika. You can serve the fajita mix in tortillas with toppings like guacamole, salsa, and a sprinkle of cheese.

Turkey Meatloaf With Mashed Sweet Potatoes

I'M A NURSE WHO HELPED CURE MY METASTIC CANCER

Turkey meatloaf is a lean and delicious alternative to traditional meatloaf. Mix ground turkey with finely chopped onions, garlic, breadcrumbs, and a blend of of your favorite herbs and spices.

Bake it until it's cooked thorough and pair it with a side of mashed sweet potatoes. Sweet potatoes are rich in vitamins A and C, providing a nutrient boost along with the comforting flavor.

I'M A NURSE WHO HELPED CURE MY METASTIC CANCER

Chicken Salad With A Twist

Get an already cooked rotisserie chicken and chop it up. Then add green leaf or romaine lettuce mixed with a variety of colorful vegetables like cherry tomatoes, cucumbers, carrots and bell peppers. You can also add a handful of spinach or arugula for an extra dose of greens. For a twist, include some fresh berries (strawberries or

I'M A NURSE WHO HELPED CURE MY METASTIC CANCER

blueberries) or Honey Crisp apples.

Finally, you can add a little extra protein by tossing in chunks of cheese (I love block Mozzarella for this), or shredded cheese. Top it off with a simple dressing.

Made in the USA
Columbia, SC
17 June 2025